W9-AUY-093

j612.63 Douglas, Ann,
DOU   1963-

         Before you were
         born.

$18.95

DATE			

GATES PUBLIC LIBRARY
1605 BUFFALO RD
ROCHESTER NY 14624

02/12/2001

BAKER & TAYLOR

Before You Were BORN

The Inside Story!

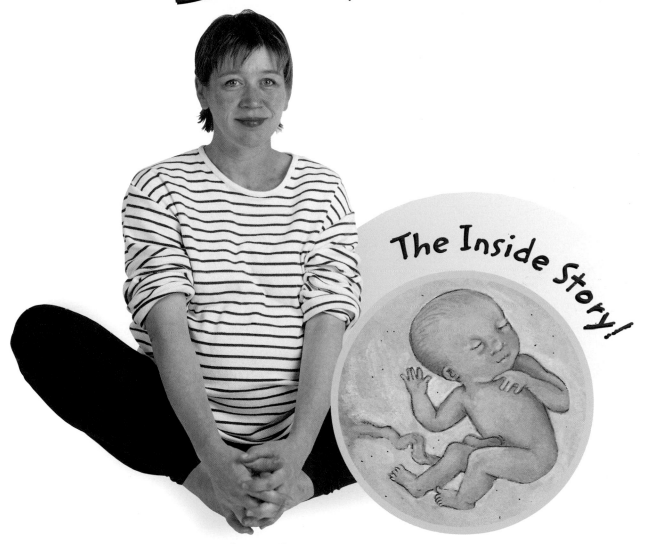

Ann Douglas

Illustrations by Eugenie Fernandes
Photographs by Gilbert Duclos

Owl

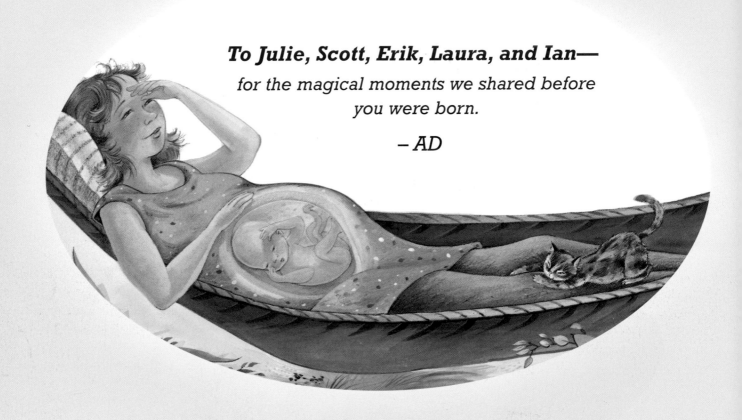

To Julie, Scott, Erik, Laura, and Ian—
for the magical moments we shared before
you were born.

– AD

CONTENTS

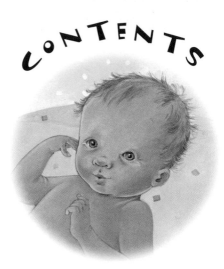

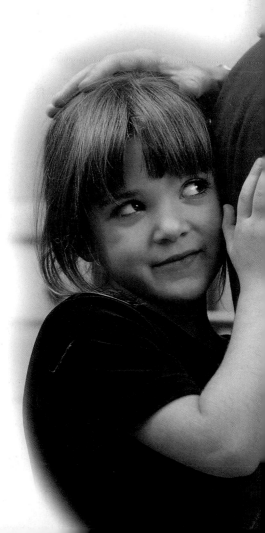

I Was That SMALL?

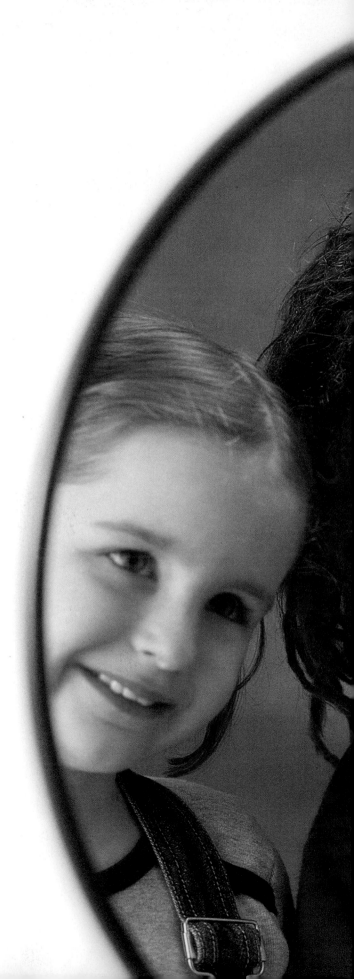

You know what you look like now. You see yourself in the mirror every day. But have you ever wondered what you looked like *before* you were born?

In the very beginning, you were round like an egg. In fact, you were an egg—a special egg inside your mother's body. The egg was special because it had joined with a sperm cell from your father's body, which meant it could grow into a human being.

It didn't have a hard shell like the eggs in your refrigerator. It was soft on the outside. Very quickly, the egg began to change. It grew by dividing itself in half over and over again until it began to look like a tiny human being. That human being was you!

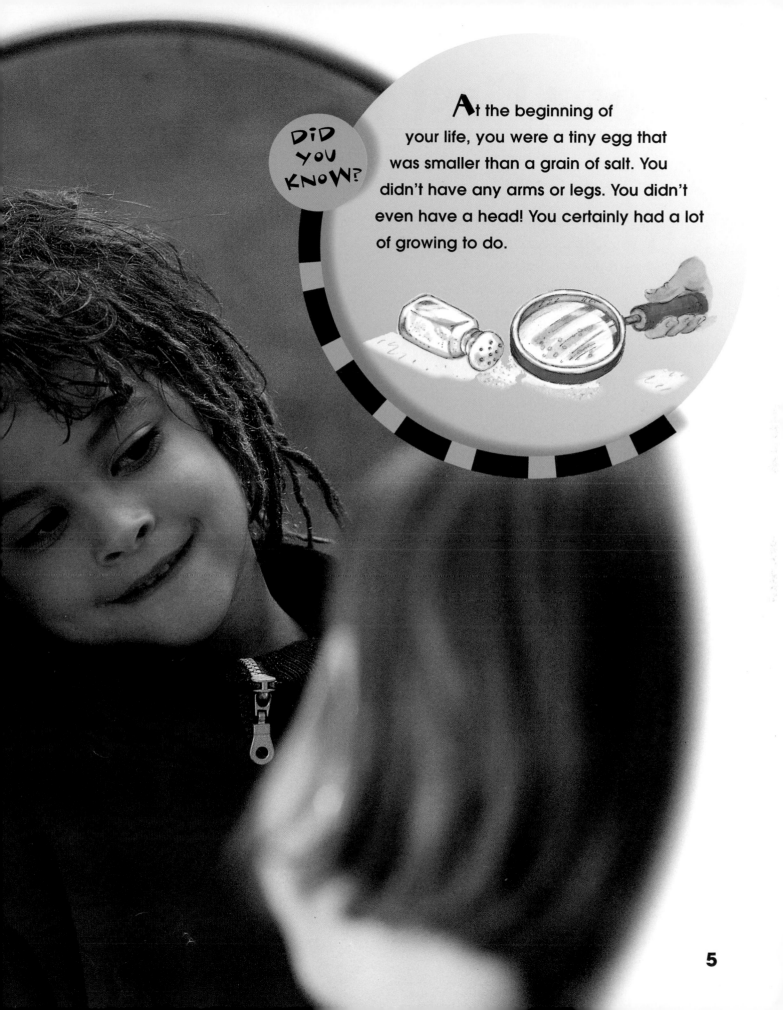

At the beginning of your life, you were a tiny egg that was smaller than a grain of salt. You didn't have any arms or legs. You didn't even have a head! You certainly had a lot of growing to do.

Your First HoME

When you were still very small, you took an exciting journey. You needed a good place to grow, so you floated down your mother's Fallopian tube and into her uterus. You attached yourself to the wall of her uterus—your home for the next nine months.

This warm, dark, wet place is the **uterus**. When you first arrived, your mother's uterus was the size of her fist. It grew bigger and bigger as you did.

BABY Science

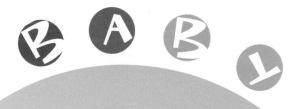

Next time you're in the bathtub, imagine what it was like to float around inside your amniotic sac—the tiny indoor swimming pool you lived in when you were growing inside your mother's body. It was dark inside the amniotic sac, so be sure to close your eyes, too!

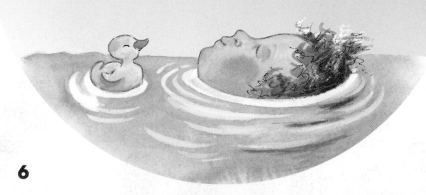

Inside the uterus is the **amniotic sac**. It was like a pillow that protected you against bumps. You floated inside, in a warm, salty liquid called amniotic fluid.

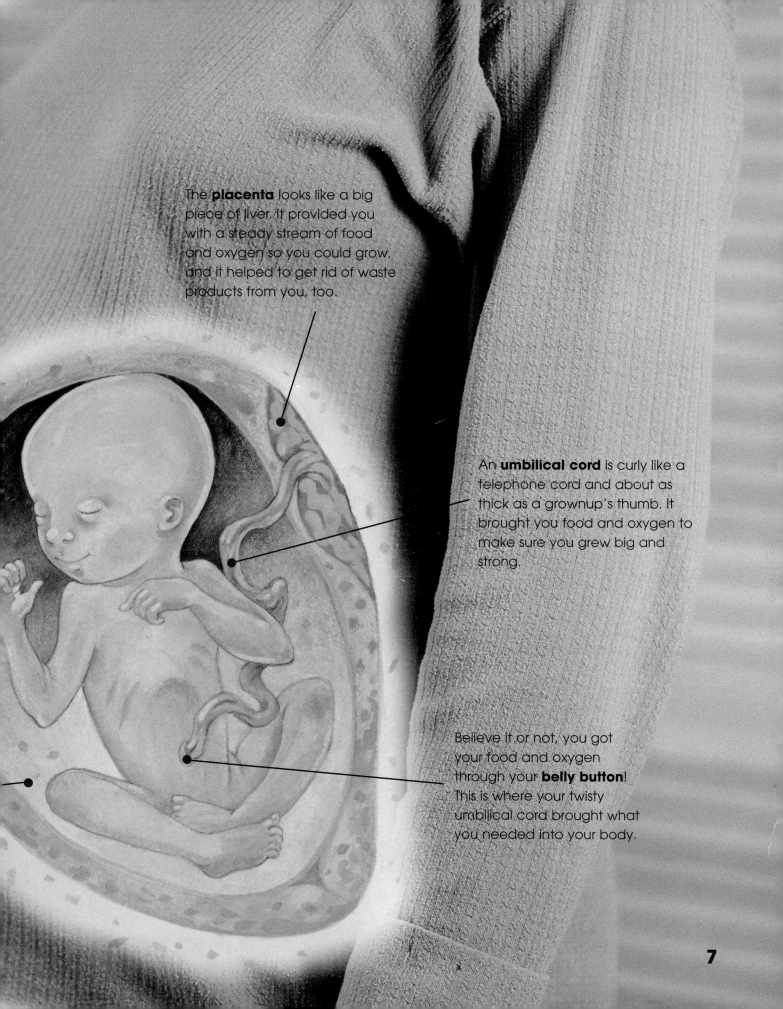

The **placenta** looks like a big piece of liver. It provided you with a steady stream of food and oxygen so you could grow, and it helped to get rid of waste products from you, too.

An **umbilical cord** is curly like a telephone cord and about as thick as a grownup's thumb. It brought you food and oxygen to make sure you grew big and strong.

Believe it or not, you got your food and oxygen through your **belly button**! This is where your twisty umbilical cord brought what you needed into your body.

That Was ME?

During your first few weeks inside your mother's body you looked more like a strange, prehistoric creature than a human being. Your bones were visible on the outside of your body. You even had a tail! Your head was larger than the rest of your body, and you had no arms or legs.

But soon, your body grew longer. Your arms started to grow. You developed hands and feet. And your tail began to disappear.

By the time you'd spent about three months inside your mother, you already had all the body parts you needed to grow into a full-sized baby. You were starting to look human, but you were still tiny. Your entire body was smaller than the size of your mother's thumb. Your job during the last six months of your mother's pregnancy was to grow and grow and grow!

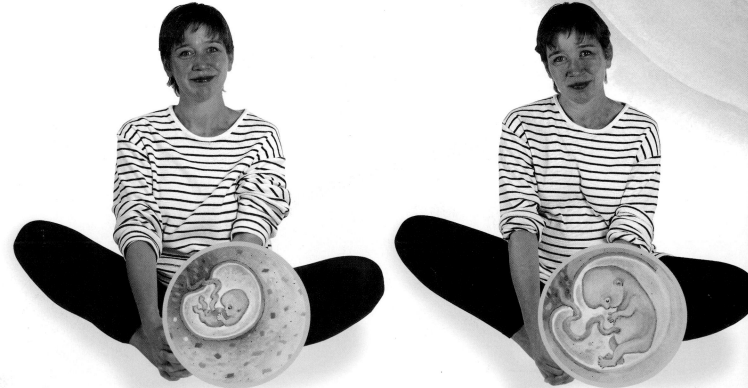

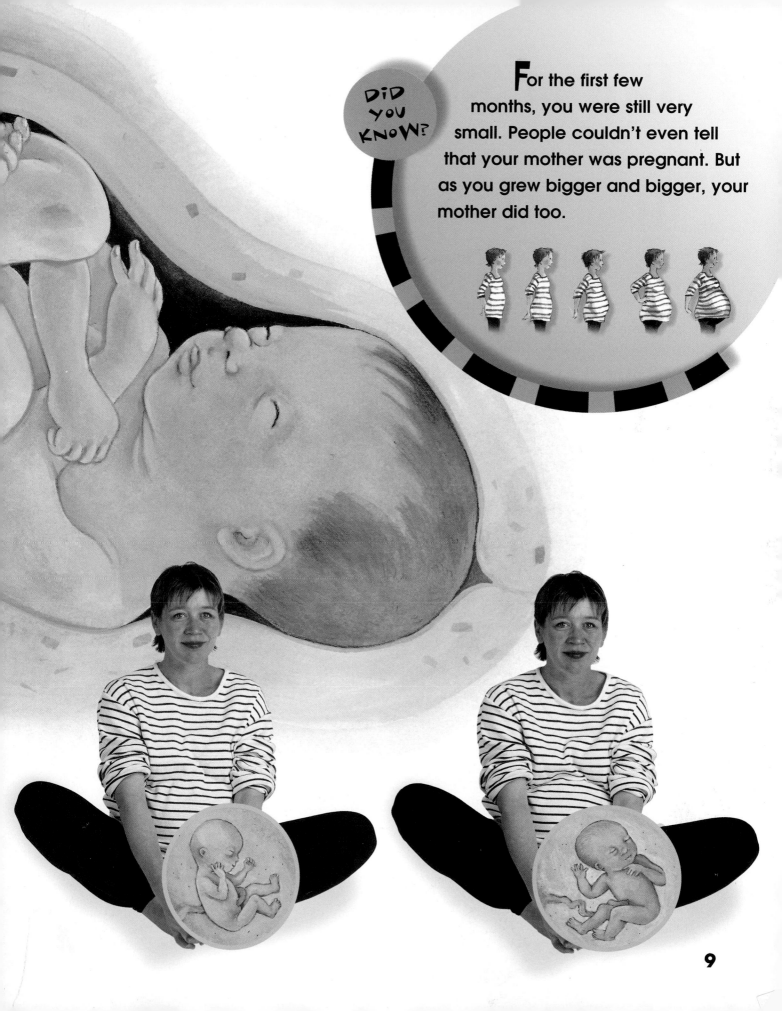

For the first few months, you were still very small. People couldn't even tell that your mother was pregnant. But as you grew bigger and bigger, your mother did too.

9

Room SERVICE!

How did you get all the food you needed to eat and the oxygen you needed to breathe to help you do all that growing?

You got most of your food and oxygen through your umbilical cord. It was attached to you at your belly button and to your mother at an organ called a placenta. The placenta took food and oxygen from your mother's bloodstream and gave them to you. The placenta also took away all the waste products your body produced. It was like a refrigerator and a toilet all in one!

The amniotic fluid you were floating in also provided you with a snack in between meals. Most of the time when you swallowed it, it just tasted salty. But if your mother ate something really spicy—like a slice of pizza with lots of garlic on it—you might have been able to taste the garlic, too.

DID YOU KNOW?

Just before you were born, you were drinking about 750 ml (3 cups) of amniotic fluid a day. That's a lot of liquid for a little baby! For the same amount of liquid, an adult would have to drink more than 60 baby bottles a day.

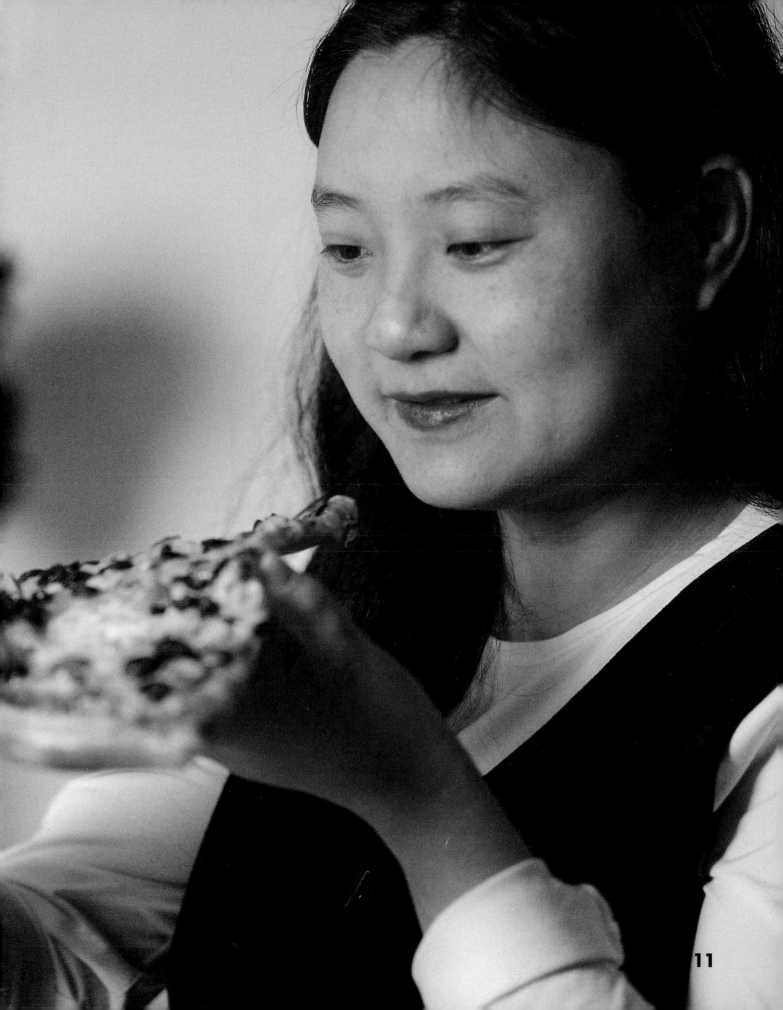

Warm FUZZIES

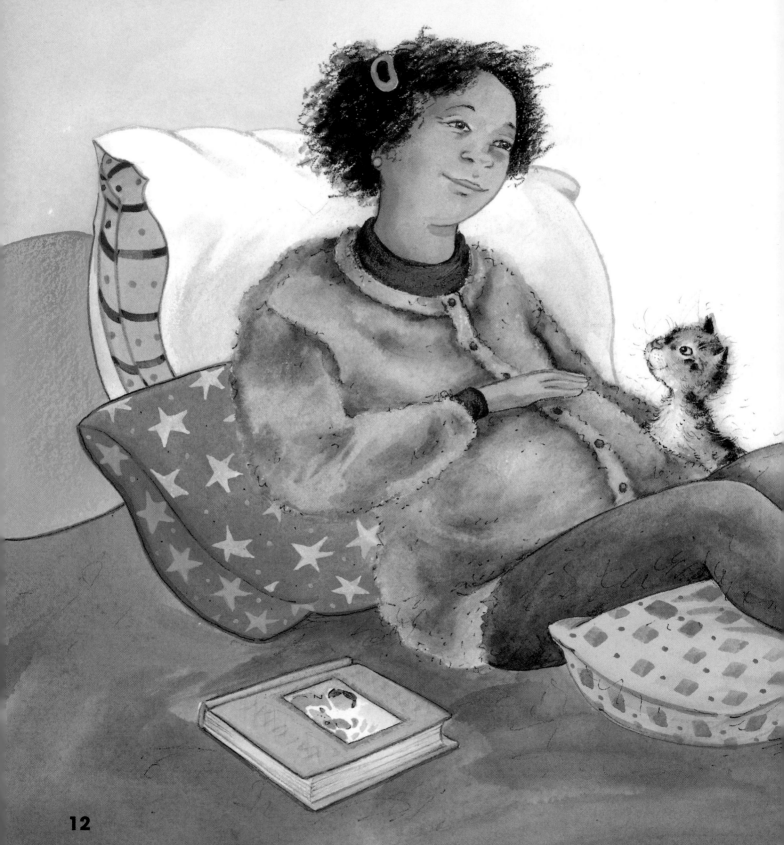

Your body was designed to keep you warm and wrinkle-free while you were inside your mother's body.

Have you ever put on so much sunscreen or hand lotion that it just gets smeared all over your skin? That is what your skin looked like, because it was coated with a slippery white layer called vernix. The vernix protected your skin from the amniotic fluid—after nine months, you'd be pretty wrinkly without it! You also had a fine layer of hair all over your body that protected you, too. It helped to keep the vernix from being washed away by the amniotic fluid.

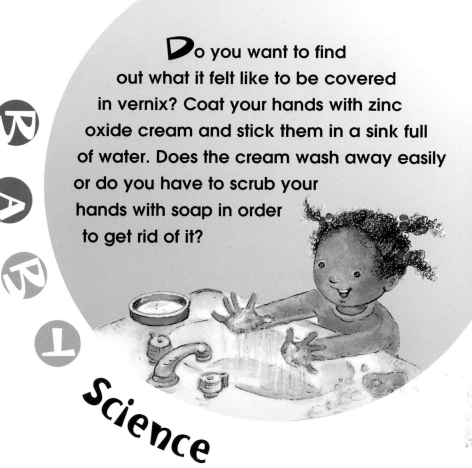

PART

Science

Do you want to find out what it felt like to be covered in vernix? Coat your hands with zinc oxide cream and stick them in a sink full of water. Does the cream wash away easily or do you have to scrub your hands with soap in order to get rid of it?

For a long time, you were very skinny. Your body was so busy getting longer and bigger that it didn't have a chance to get chubby. A month or two before you were born, your body started to build up a layer of fat. This would help to keep you warm after you left your warm, cozy home inside your mother's body.

On the MOVE!

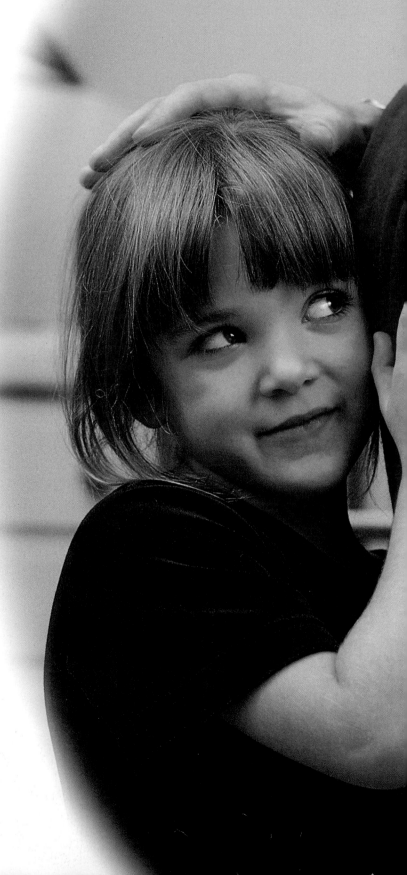

You moved around a lot before you were born. At first your mother felt as if a goldfish was swimming around, or a butterfly was fluttering, inside her. When you were still very tiny, you could do entire somersaults in your mother's uterus. You were doing baby gymnastics!

As you grew bigger and stronger, your mother felt as if a small animal, like a bunny, was bumping and squirming around inside her. She could even feel tiny jabs from your baby hands and feet. Not only could your mother feel these kicks, sometimes she could even see them!

When your mother felt you moving around, she would sit still, put her hand on her stomach, and think how excited she was about meeting you one day soon. In the last few months of her pregnancy, when other people touched her stomach, they could feel you moving around, too. Your kicks had grown that strong!

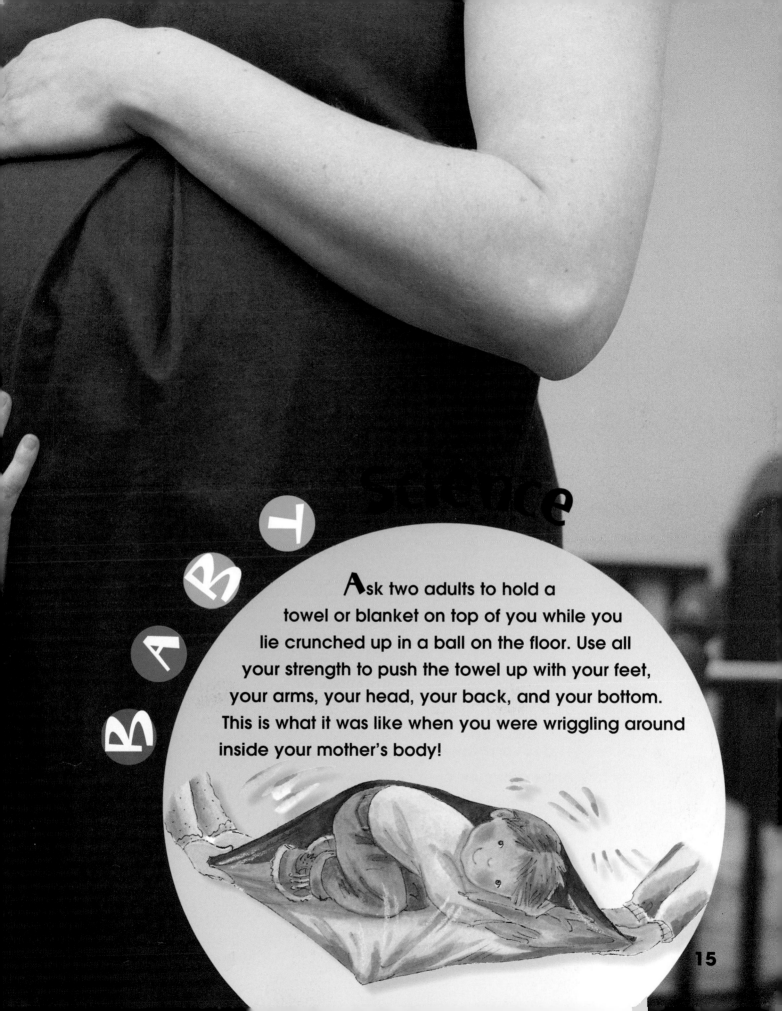

BABY Science

Ask two adults to hold a towel or blanket on top of you while you lie crunched up in a ball on the floor. Use all your strength to push the towel up with your feet, your arms, your head, your back, and your bottom. This is what it was like when you were wriggling around inside your mother's body!

Baby at PLAY

You didn't have toys inside your mother's body, so what did you do all day?

Well, you kept your hands busy. Sometimes you grabbed your umbilical cord. You rubbed your face and sucked your thumb. You could get your thumb in your mouth even though you couldn't see what you were doing. In fact, you were better at it than you were just after you were born. Maybe you were so used to sucking your thumb in the dark, you became confused when you could actually see it!

feet

head

DID YOU KNOW?

Until a few years ago, scientists could only guess what babies were doing in their mothers' bodies. Today, scientists use a special machine known as an ultrasound. Ultrasound machines send soundwaves through the mother's body and draw a picture on a TV screen (like the one above) that lets doctors see what the unborn baby is doing. Sometimes the doctor can even tell if it's a boy or a girl.

16

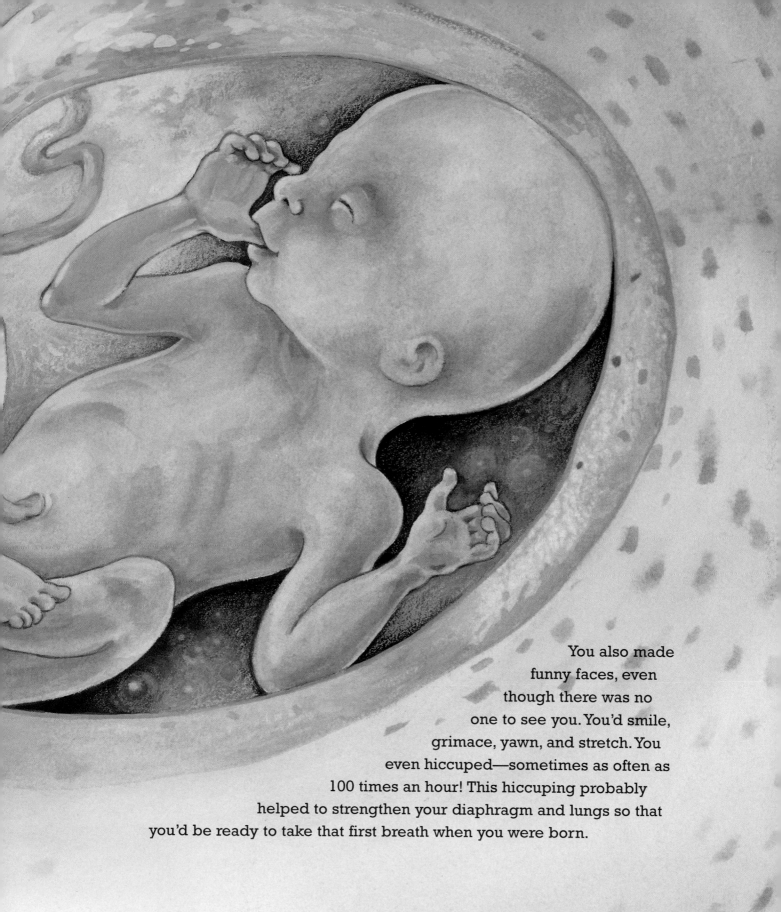

You also made
funny faces, even
though there was no
one to see you. You'd smile,
grimace, yawn, and stretch. You
even hiccuped—sometimes as often as
100 times an hour! This hiccuping probably
helped to strengthen your diaphragm and lungs so that
you'd be ready to take that first breath when you were born.

Napping on the RUN

When you were inside your mother's body, you spent a lot more time sleeping than awake. You only woke up for a couple of minutes at a time.

It's no wonder you were so sleepy. Your body was working hard to grow big and strong. As your mother went about her day, walking around the house, going to work, or doing the grocery shopping, her movements gently rocked you to sleep.

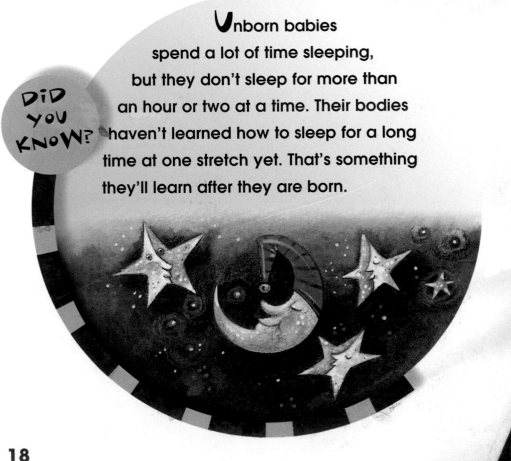

DID YOU KNOW?

Unborn babies spend a lot of time sleeping, but they don't sleep for more than an hour or two at a time. Their bodies haven't learned how to sleep for a long time at one stretch yet. That's something they'll learn after they are born.

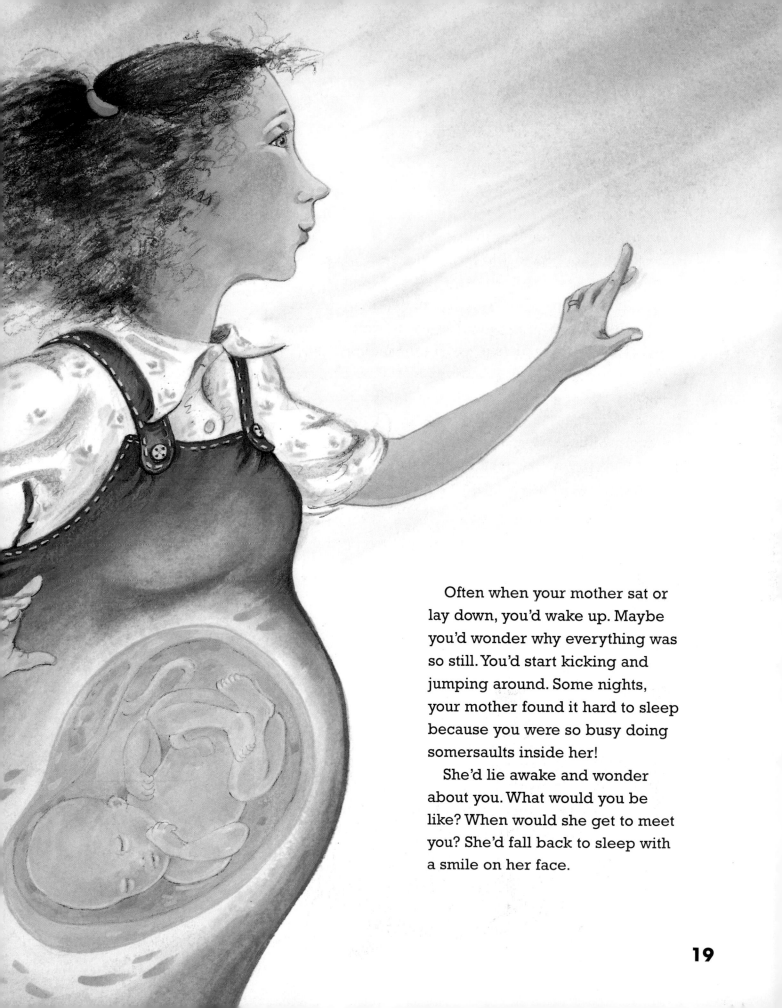

Often when your mother sat or lay down, you'd wake up. Maybe you'd wonder why everything was so still. You'd start kicking and jumping around. Some nights, your mother found it hard to sleep because you were so busy doing somersaults inside her!

She'd lie awake and wonder about you. What would you be like? When would she get to meet you? She'd fall back to sleep with a smile on her face.

What's Up, Doc?

You started visiting the doctor long before you were born. In fact, you had your first checkup when you were no bigger than your mother's thumb!

Each time your mother went for a checkup, the doctor or midwife measured her belly to see how much her uterus had grown. The measurement told her that you were growing, too. Your mother was also weighed, to see how much weight the two of you were gaining.

The doctor or midwife used a special type of stethoscope called a doppler to listen to your heartbeat. It made a very fast swooshing noise as it echoed across the room. Swoosh-swoosh-swoosh. Sometimes you'd wriggle away and the doctor or midwife would have to find you and start listening all over again.

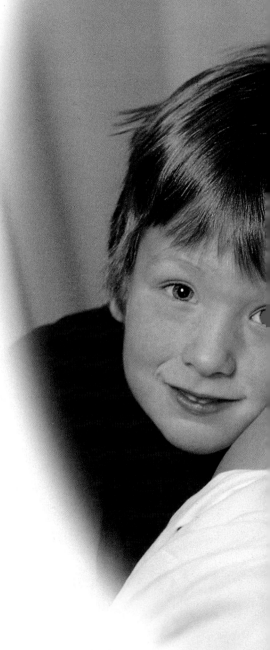

DID YOU KNOW?

Your little heart was hard at work pumping blood through you to feed your growing body when you were inside your mother. An unborn baby's heart beats twice as fast as its mother's heart beats.

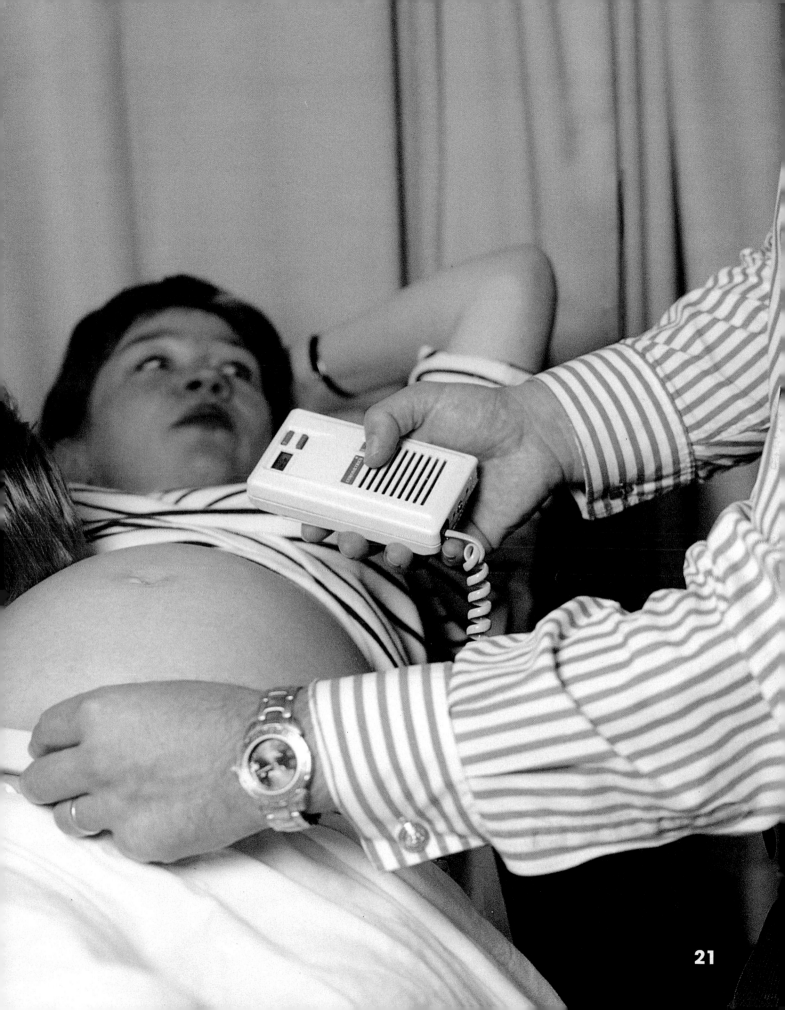

I SPY!

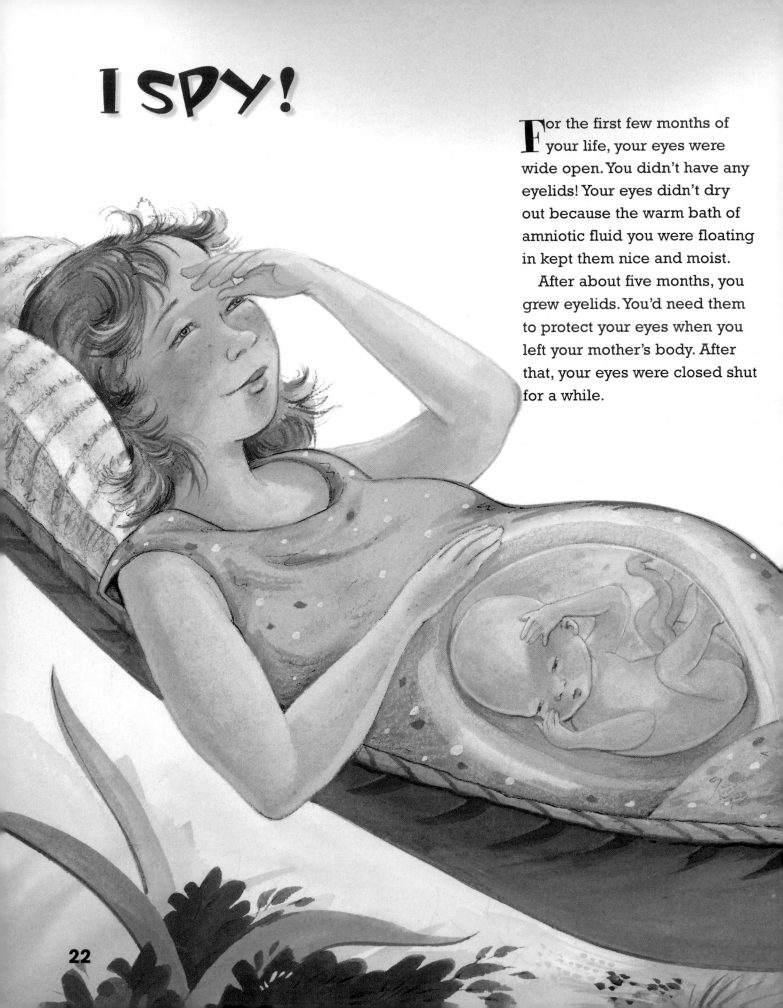

For the first few months of your life, your eyes were wide open. You didn't have any eyelids! Your eyes didn't dry out because the warm bath of amniotic fluid you were floating in kept them nice and moist.

After about five months, you grew eyelids. You'd need them to protect your eyes when you left your mother's body. After that, your eyes were closed shut for a while.

A few months before you were ready to be born, your eyes opened up again. You couldn't see clearly, but you could tell the difference between light and dark. If the sun or another bright light was shining on your mother's stomach, you might have even turned your head so the bright light wouldn't shine right in your eyes. Maybe you were looking for a pair of sunglasses!

Here's how to see what unborn babies see when their mothers are out on a sunny day. Take a flashlight into a dark room. Spread your fingers and hold your hand up so your knuckles are facing you. Turn the flashlight on and place it behind the thin piece of skin that runs between your thumb and index finger (the one you use to point). The light shining through your skin is similar to what an unborn baby sees.

Science

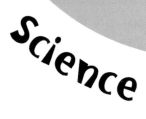

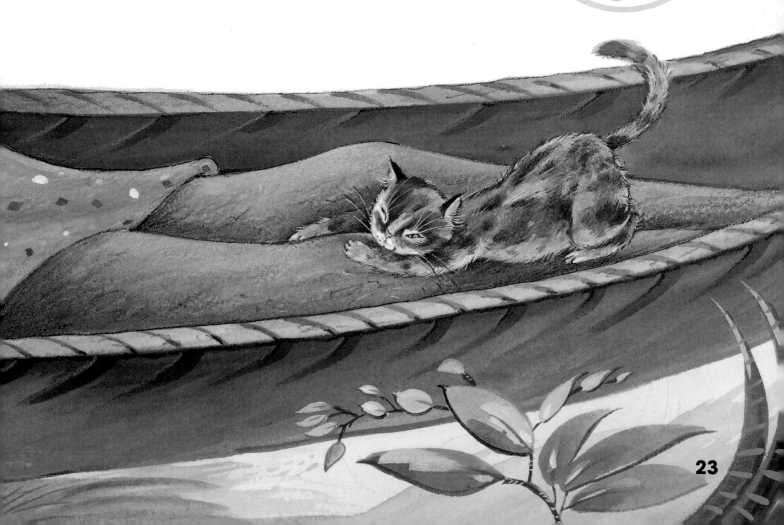

23

HEAR This

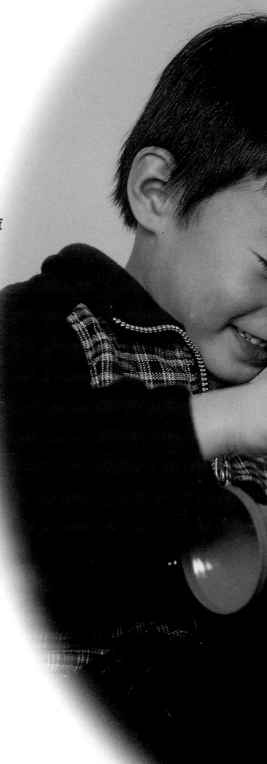

You probably think your home before you were born was nice and quiet. In fact, your mother's body made all kinds of sounds. And, by the time you were six months old, you could certainly use your ears! You heard the sound of her heart pumping blood through her body, her lungs emptying and filling with air, the blood swishing through her large blood vessels, her stomach digesting food, and her intestines getting rid of waste. It's amazing you got any sleep with all that noise!

You also heard sounds from *outside* your mother's body. Sometimes loud bangs startled you, and your mother could feel you jump. You heard your mother's voice and the voices of other people in your family: your father, your grandparents, and your brothers and sisters. That's why you already knew their voices when you were born.

BABY Science

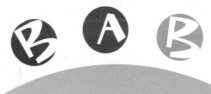

Listen to the swishing sounds that a dishwasher makes. That's the type of sound that you heard all the time when you were growing inside your mother's body.

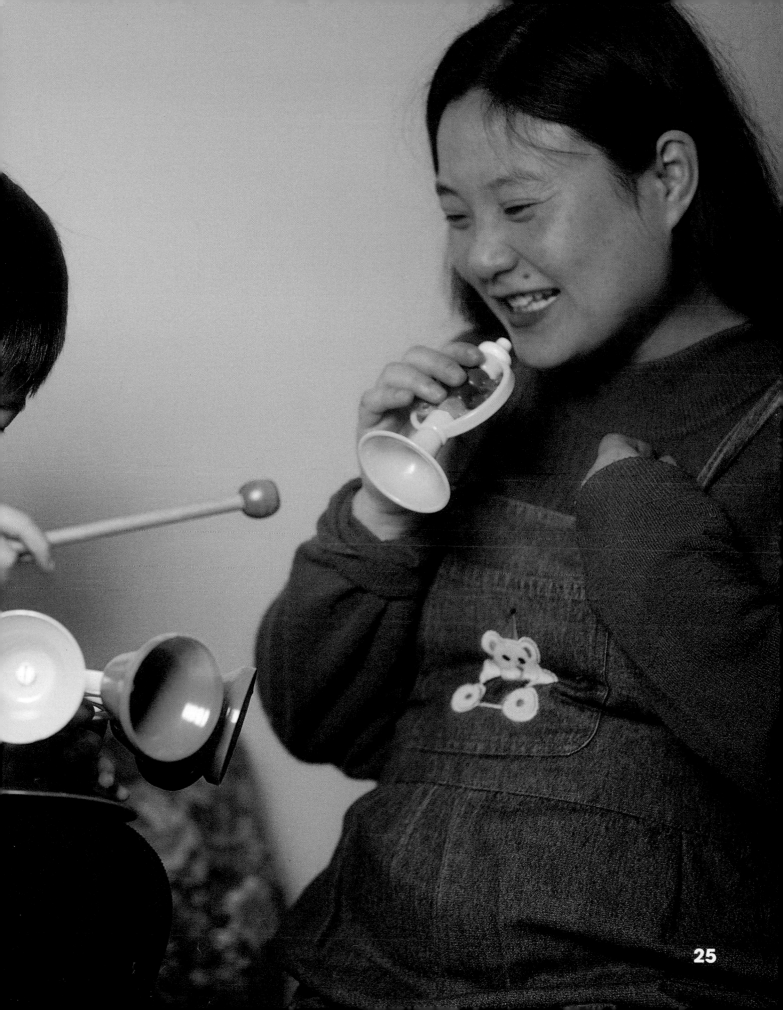

Womb MATES

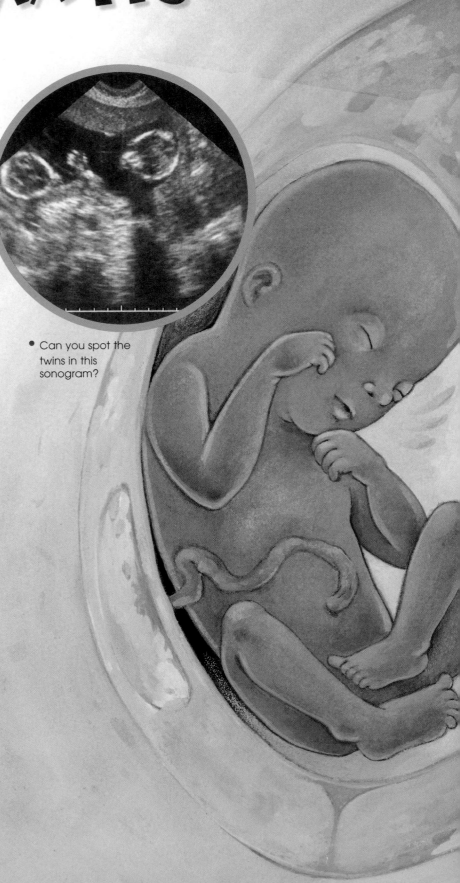

Most of the time, pregnant women have one baby growing in their uterus at a time. But, sometimes, they may have two or even more.

When two babies are growing together in one uterus, they are called twins. Sometimes twins come from the same egg. These are called identical twins because they look almost exactly the same. Twins that come from two different eggs are called fraternal twins. They don't look any more alike than other brothers and sisters.

Some families have three babies, called triplets, or four (quadruplets), or even more at the same time. Imagine how many diapers that would be to change!

• Can you spot the twins in this sonogram?

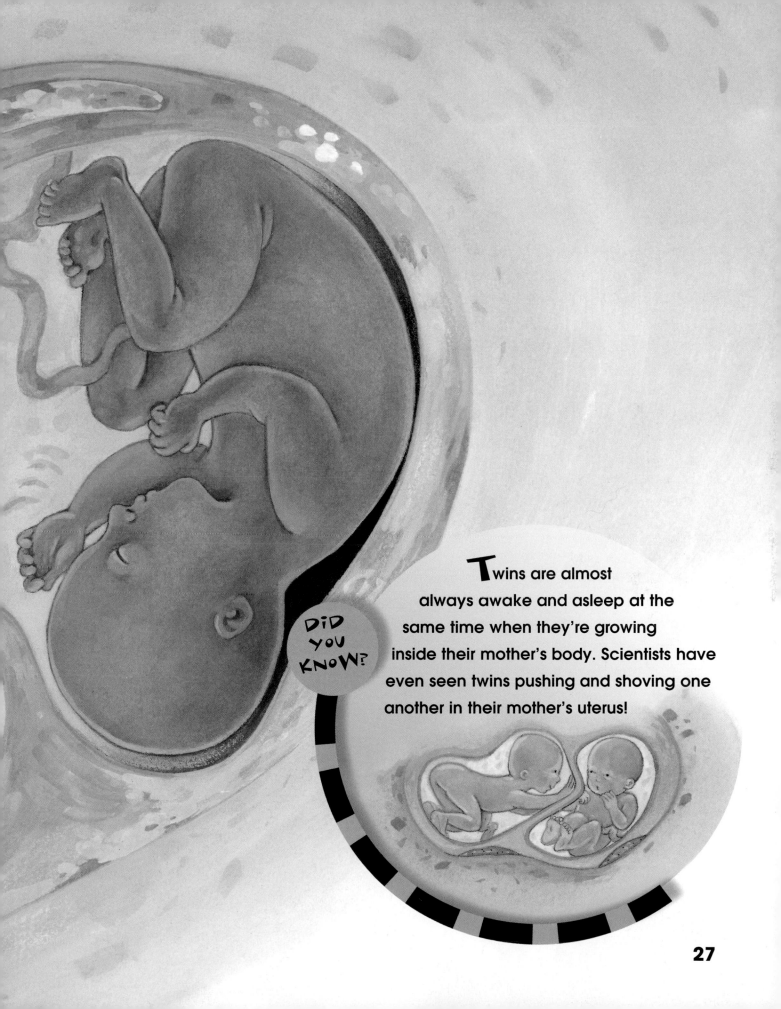

DID YOU KNOW?

Twins are almost always awake and asleep at the same time when they're growing inside their mother's body. Scientists have even seen twins pushing and shoving one another in their mother's uterus!

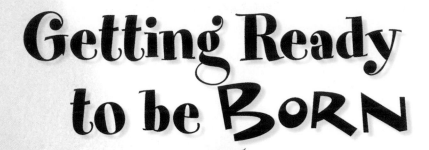

Getting Ready to be BORN

After about nine months, you'd done all the growing you could do inside your mother's body. In fact, you were getting so big there was hardly any room to move around at all! You were finally ready to leave your first home.

Your parents and the rest of your family were very excited about meeting you. Everybody knew the big day was coming, but no one knew exactly when you were going to be born. The doctor or midwife tried to figure it out. Your parents tried to guess. Even the people your mother met in the grocery store tried to guess.

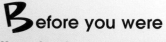

Before you were born, the doctor or midwife had to figure out if your head was pointing up (this would make your birth more difficult) or down toward your mother's feet (the way it was supposed to be pointing). Try out your baby detective skills! Put a doll in a pillowcase and try to figure out which way it's facing. Too easy? Try wrapping the doll in a towel or blanket first.

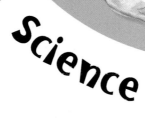

In the end, it was something inside you that decided when it was time for you to leave the warm, cozy spot inside your mother's body. And when you were ready, you sent a signal to your mother's brain telling her that it was time to have a baby. Your birth day had arrived!

Happy Birthday, BABY!

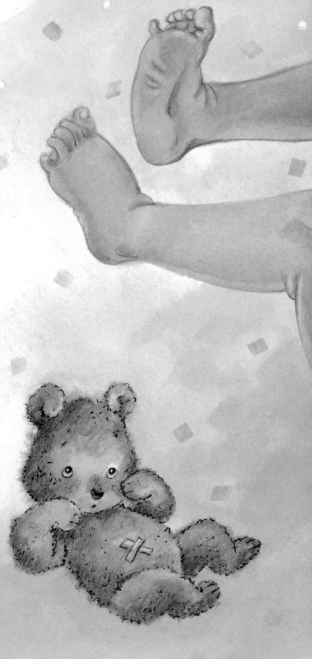

When you sent that special signal that it was time for you to be born, your mother's body got ready. Her uterus began to tighten so it could open up the passageway leading out of her body. Her body worked very hard to push you through the birth canal and out of her. Just when she was getting very tired, suddenly there you were: the baby she had been wanting to hold for nine months!

You took your first breath. You let out a tiny cry that helped to clear the mucus from your throat and mouth. The doctor or midwife put you on your mother's stomach and you tried to wiggle your way up to one of her breasts to have a drink. You were only seconds old, but you were already very smart.

You looked at the amazing world around you. At first you were a little frightened, but then you heard your mother's and father's voices, and you felt safe. Your parents held you and looked right into your eyes. "Happy birthday, baby," they said. "Welcome to the world!"

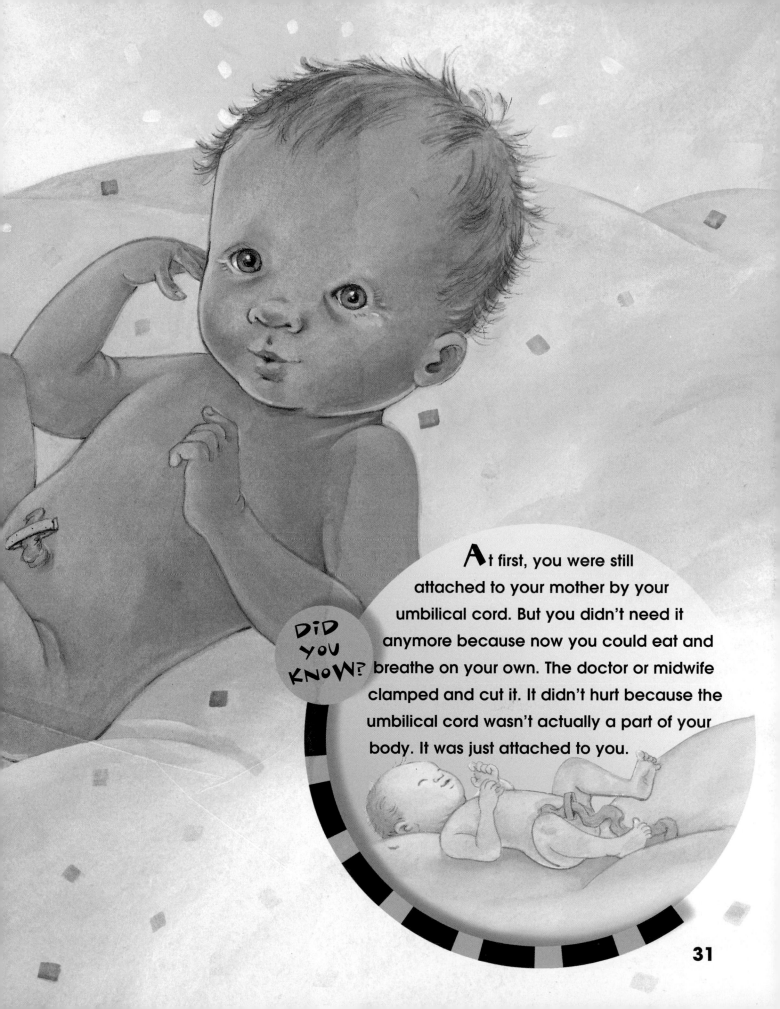

DID **YOU** **KNOW?**

At first, you were still attached to your mother by your umbilical cord. But you didn't need it anymore because now you could eat and breathe on your own. The doctor or midwife clamped and cut it. It didn't hurt because the umbilical cord wasn't actually a part of your body. It was just attached to you.

Owl Books are published by Greey de Pencier Books Inc.
70 The Esplanade, Suite 400, Toronto, Ontario M5E 1R2

The Owl colophon is a trademark of Owl Children's Trust Inc.
Greey de Pencier Books Inc. is a licensed user of trademarks of Owl Children's Trust Inc.

Text © 2000 Ann Douglas
Illustrations © 2000 Eugenie Fernandes
Photographs © 2000 Gilbert Duclos

All rights reserved. No part of this book may be reproduced or copied in any form without
written consent from the publisher.

Distributed in the United States by Firefly Books (U.S.) Inc.
230 Fifth Avenue, Suite 1607, New York, NY 10001

We acknowledge the financial support of the Canada Council for the Arts, the Ontario
Arts Council, and the Government of Canada through the Book Publishing Industry
Development Program (BPIDP) for our publishing activities.

Cataloguing in Publication Data

Douglas, Ann, 1963–
        Before you were born : the inside story!

ISBN 1-894379-01-2 (bound)   ISBN 1-894379-02-0 (pbk.)

1. Pregnancy — Juvenile literature. 2. Embryology, Human — Juvenile literature.
I. Fernandes, Eugenie, 1943–   . II. Title.

RG525.5.D68   2000   j612.6'3   C00-930697-8

Design & art direction: **Word & Image Design Studio Inc.**
Illustrations: **Eugenie Fernandes**
All photos by **Gilbert Duclos,** except sonograms on pages 16 and 26, courtesy
of **Amy Pinchuk**

The activities in this book have been tested, and are safe when conducted as instructed.
The publisher accepts no responsibility for any damage caused or sustained due to the
use or misuse of ideas or materials featured herein.

Printed in Hong Kong

A   B   C   D   E   F

0177

PLEASE SHARE YOUR THOUGHTS ON THIS BOOK

comments:	comments:
comments:	comments:
comments:	comments:
comments:	comments:
comments:	comments:
comments:	comments: